VEGAN COOKING BEGINNERS

EVERYDAY EASY AND HEALTHY VEGAN RECIPES

By David D. Kings

Copyrights 2017 David D. Kings

No part of this book can be transmitted or reproduced in any form including print, electronic, photocopying, scanning, mechanical or recording without prior written permission from the author.

All information, ideas, and guidelines presented here are for educational purposes only. This book cannot be used to replace information provided with the device. All readers are encouraged to seek professional advice when needed.

TABLE OF CONTENTS

INTRODUCTION 1
   BECOME A VEGETARIAN AND ENJOY THE VARIOUS BENEFITS! 1
   USING SIMPLE VEGAN RECIPES TO BENEFIT YOUR WALLET, HEALTH AND BODY 5
   MAKE USE OF EASY VEGAN RECIPES TO BENEFIT YOUR BANK ACCOUNT, HEALTH, AND BODY 6

CHAPTER 1 9
   RAW VEGAN RECIPES 9
   WHY SIMPLE RAW VEGAN RECIPES CAN GIVE RADIANT HEALTH 9
   THERE ARE MANY OTHER HEALTH BENEFITS OF EATING RAW 10
   ALTER YOUR LIFESTYLE, NOT THE DIET 10
   HIGH-PROTEIN DIETS DON'T HAVE TO INCLUDE MEAT 11
   WHAT FOODS CAN I PUT INTO MY RAW VEGAN RECIPES? 11

CHAPTER 2 13
   EASY AND HEALTHY VEGAN BREAKFAST RECIPES 13
   SOUTIIWEST SCRAMBLE WITH GREENS (TOFU) 13
   PROTEIN OAT BOWL 15
   BREAKFAST BURRITOS 16

MAPLE GINGER PANCAKES..19
CHOCOLATE CHIP, APRICOT, AND ORANGE SCONES…21
POMEGRANATE QUINOA PORRIDGE.................................24
STEWED APPLES..25
CHEWY HOMEMADE GRANOLA BARS (GLUTEN FREE) 27

CHAPTER 3..30
EASY AND HEALTHY VEGAN LUNCH RECIPES..............30
MEXICAN AVOCADO SALAD..30
CRAZY DELICIOUS RAW PAD THAI...................................31
KALE & WILD RICE STIR FLY..32
EXTRA CREAMY MAC AND CHEESE.................................33
GRILLED BUFFALO TOFU PO' BOY WITH APPLE SLAW 35
MEXICAN BLACK BEAN SOUP...36
CRAB CAKES WITH SWEET BALSAMIC MAYO...............38
CRISPY TOFU NUGGETS..40
BLACK BEAN VEGAN WRAPS..42
SOUTHWESTERN VEGAN GRILLED CHEESE SANDWICH 43

CHAPTER 4..45
EASY AND HEALTHY VEGAN DINNER RECIPES.............45
ZUCCHINI PASTA WITH PESTO SAUCE...........................48
TEMPEH FISH N CHIPS W/ TARTAR SAUCE....................50
VEGAN MUSHROOM STROGANOFF.................................53
THE VEGAN EGGPLANT CRUNCHBURGER.....................54

BALSAMIC BBQ SEITAN AND TEMPEH RIBS...................58
TACOS SIN CARNE..67
PASTA WITH FRESH TOMATO SAUCE...............................69

INTRODUCTION

Vegan Recipes have amazing nutritional value and can have marvelous and incredible results on the body providing essential nutrients to your body. They boost your energy and you can experience some life-changing benefits such as weight loss, clearer and vibrant skin, free of some common heart diseases, no blood pressure etc.

BECOME A VEGETARIAN AND ENJOY THE VARIOUS BENEFITS!

- Vegetarian recipes such as oat yogurt, green salads, tomato salad, raw whole grain muesli, vegetables soup provide essential proteins, carbohydrates, vitamins, fiber, and minerals.

- They have no preservatives, no additives and also no oil.

- Generally they are broiled or boiled which is very good for health as then the food becomes oil free containing all the necessary nutrients.

- They taste delicious and at the same time provide nutrition and are useful in reducing cholesterol and other health alarming diseases.

- They help in reducing extra calories and you can stay fit and healthy while having these recipes.

- Vegan baking is another option, if you want to make your food oil free.

They have become extremely popular as they possess various advantages and they help in assisting various people suffering from alarming diseases in staying fit and fine.

You can also have fun and can enjoy having vegan recipes by going to healthy vacations. There are many benefits of adopting a vegetarian diet as it gives the energy and all the necessary nutrients also. It is available in different varieties giving you ample of choices to choose one according to your taste.

They can be made quickly and you should keep various things in mind while making a vegetarian recipe. It should be made using the things which contain low fat content, use less sugar and whole foods should be used more.

Fatty things should be avoided and you should always try to replace the things containing fat with raw, healthy and oil free things.

Sugar can be replaced by various substitutes of sugar or sweeteners like sucanat or maple syrup; as they break down and get absorbed into the blood stream much slower than the normal white sugar. Various fruits can also be used as they contain natural sweetness which is not harmful to health and body. Thus we can maintain the blood sugar balance in our body in easier manner.

Whole foods should be included in the recipes in their natural state, so that they do not loose their essential components. Whole wheat flour instead of white; sucanat, brown rice syrup or maple syrup instead of white sugar, and coconut oil instead of butter or margarine should be used in making healthier and yummy recipes.

Our body other than proteins and carbohydrates also need a good amount of vitamins and minerals. Researches have shown that fruits and vegetables are full of minerals,vitamins,carbohydrates and fiber. Vegan food recipes are great for health as they have neither preservatives nor additives nor it is fried in oil. They are normally broiled or boiled. Some vegan recipes are oat yogurt,green salads,tomato salad,raw whole grain muesli,vegetables soup. Vegan food recipes are trouble-free and quick to cook. People suffering from health alarming diseases and high cholesterol are recommended to have only greens. That is why vegan food recipes are known to be useful and healthy.

Vegan food recipes moreover help to lose those added kilos. If you are round or overweight and are hunting out for a healthy diet regime, what could be more useful than having vegan recipes and raw food. And in 1 week you be able to reap the results. You can go on for a extended period if you wish for to stay fit and healthy. But if you are not strong mentally and yearn for non-vegetarian food then you can never go on on vegan meals for a long time. Vegan recipes have gotten extremely popular and there's two divergent views concerning it. Lots of fitness and nutritionists consider that vegan food recipes assists one to stay healthy and fit and is a good means to reduce cholesterol and fat. Others feel vegan recipes are overestimated and are in reality not best for our body - the argument is that human body requires quite a bit of protein that a vegan diet can't offer enough. Again, not everybody can consume veg centered dishes all the time.

Vegetarians generally go for foods like beets, apples, raw grains, carrots, oats, rye, almonds, sesame seeds, oranges, pumpkins, asparagus, tomatoes, red peppers, broccoli, buckwheat, spinach, cabbages, pomegranate, etc. It's been observed that majority of folks that resolutely follow a vegan diet plan are rather lean and fat free with lower sugar, BP and cholesterol.

It is commonly accepted that adequate health is almost fail-safe if you do regular work-outs backed by a good veg diet plan. Many of the Yoga preachers adhere to a vegan food regimen which is one of the reasons why they stay slim and healthy. Conversely, since vegetarian diet is devoid of proteins it will not assist in building muscle groups and strength. If you are a muscle builder, then a regular protein diet is mandatory and meat and eggs are a good protein source. Some prefer to keep semi-vegan to benefit from the facets of both worlds. Salads may be combined with bacon strips and chicken breast, but its important to keep away from fried meat. Meat or chicken kebabs might be a decent choice once in a while as they're prepared free of oil. The plan is to remain mostly vegetarian and use oil free baked chicken breast ever so often.

USING SIMPLE VEGAN RECIPES TO BENEFIT YOUR WALLET, HEALTH AND BODY

There are a lot of misconceptions that come with a vegan diet and lifestyle. For starters, there are a whole host of benefits for eating healthy, following a vegan diet, and utilizing the best vegan recipes. However, the main misconception is that eating vegan is instantly healthy. This is not always the case. Balance and simple recipes are of the utmost importance when it comes to a vegan lifestyle. Technically you could indulge in an entire bag of potato chips at every meal and still be considering a vegan. But you probably already know that is the opposite of healthy eating. So what can you do in order to be sure you go about your lifestyle the right way? The best starting point is to seek out the best simple recipes and the best vegan recipes.

Having a variety of the best simple vegan recipes on hand can do wonders for your diet plan and your overall health. Being a vegan comes with some temptations that are sure to surround you at all times. If you are not aware of the healthy balanced options available then you are very likely to give in and opt for fast, easy choices that can leave your heart, and your waistline, suffering later on. Push temptation to the side and take advantage of the best simple recipes and you will feel better in no time, and your heart will thank you later on.

Most people will tell you that a vegan diet that is healthy, full of fiber, and low in fat can do wonders for your heart. But as you already know, following an efficient diet such as that is easier said than done. If you can utilize some of the best vegan recipes that you can find online then your chances of engaging in a healthy and satisfying diet plan will improve greatly.

Being a vegan goes a lot deeper than simply staying clear of animal products. There is so much temptation when it comes to convenient foods, but you need to remember that these convenient, fast foods can often be the highest in fat and calories. However that does not always have to be the case. By finding the best simple foods, you can indulge in delicious meals that are easy to make and easy on your body. Isn't that exactly what you were looking for when you decided to become a vegan in the first place?

The most important thing that you should take away from this article is that a vegan lifestyle is more than just a simple choice. To truly eat healthy and benefit from the best vegan recipes you need to be committed and prepared. Many people that choose to turn to a vegan diet have no idea how to get started or how to improve their diet. By taking the time to browse through the best simple recipes and find balanced meals that suit your tastes, your budget, and your waistline you can do wonders for your overall health.

MAKE USE OF EASY VEGAN RECIPES TO BENEFIT YOUR BANK ACCOUNT, HEALTH, AND BODY

There are plenty of misunderstandings that take place with a vegan regimen and way of life. For starters, there are a whole host of benefits for eating nutritiously, abiding by a vegan diet, and choosing the best vegan recipes. However the major misunderstanding is that eating vegan is instantly a healthy thing. This is not always the situation since stability and finding good recipes are very critical when it comes to a vegan way of life. In theory you could indulge in a complete bag of potato chips at every meal and still be thought of as a vegan. But you most likely already understand that is the flip-side to healthy eating, so what standard should you be using? The best starting point is to seek out the best simple recipes and the best vegan recipes.

Having an assortment of online recipes on hand can be extremely beneficial for your diet strategy and your healthy road map. Being a vegan comes with a number of enticing means that are certain to regularly question your discipline. If you are unaware of the better balanced choices at your disposal, then you will be more inclined to surrender and choose for fast, simple choices that can leave your health, and your body, suffering later on. Put temptation over and take advantage of the simple online recipes and you will feel in no time, and your heart will appreciate you later on.

Most professionals in the health department will support the notion that a proper diet that is full of fiber and low in fat is a recipe for success but as expected, following a proficient diet such as that is hard to do. Having attainable goals is very important when it comes to planning out your strategy. The chances of whether or not you'll succeed depend highly on how motivated you stay and how mentally tough you are..

It takes more than merely not eating meat to being a vegetarian. There is a great deal of temptation when it comes to fatty foods, but you need to remember that these quick, drive through menus can often be the greatest in fat and calories. However, that does not always have to be the case. If you use logic and sensibility, you'd be able to simply determine the healthy foods from the destructive ones. By using the best online food recipes, you can indulge in appetizing dishes that are easy to make and healthy for your body.

The most essential component that you should take away from this post is that a vegan lifestyle is more than just a simple choice. To absolutely eat healthy and take advantage of good vegan recipes available to you, you need to be disciplined and willing. Many people who choose to turn to a vegan diet have no clue how to begin or how to improve their diet. Consuming healthy meals from simple food recipes will undoubtedly increase your physical and mental status. Ensuring that you consistently choose the best food recipes and being consistent with your diet are important factors for your overall health.

CHAPTER 1

RAW VEGAN RECIPES

Preparing simple raw vegan recipes can be surprisingly pleasurable. There are hundreds of simple recipes and the list of raw vegan ingredients to choose from is amazing. A full wholesome meal of entrees, soups, salads, desserts, smoothies and drinks can be created using simple raw vegan recipes. It will taste fantastic and give your health a massive boost.

WHY SIMPLE RAW VEGAN RECIPES CAN GIVE RADIANT HEALTH

All the goodness and nutrients naturally present in food are found in Raw Vegan recipes.

Cooking above 130 degrees damages or destroys the vitamins and nutrients, which are required by the body. It's like eating empty foods, or empty calories, that just fill you up temporarily.

Your skin will feel and looks cleaner and the need for moisturiser becomes a lot less. The natural health from the raw food transfers to your body and skin. Your hair will also benefit and look a lot more naturally shiny & healthy.

Imagine watering a plant. Give it fresh water with nutrients each day and the leaves will shine and the flowers will blossom. You give it soapy dishwater to drink instead, and it will soon appear unhealthy.

THERE ARE MANY OTHER HEALTH BENEFITS OF EATING RAW

The Raw food diet has helped many people find health when nothing else did. It can give healthy levels of blood cholesterol and blood sugar levels, pain-free joints, a permanent boost to your immune system, amazingly restful sleep and unbelievable energy.

ALTER YOUR LIFESTYLE, NOT THE DIET

Replacing fatty and dairy products from recipes is perhaps the first step towards healthier eating. Your body probably requires four times less energy to digest raw food over processed food, and the supplementary energy is freed up to make you feel a lot more alive. Cellulite disappears, weight is lost, headaches disappear.

Diets cause distress to your body. Most diets have short term benefits, at best, but don't address the problem long term. Diets make you less healthy since the weight loss that occurs on these diets is caused by bodily distress, not healthy living.

HIGH-PROTEIN DIETS DON'T HAVE TO INCLUDE MEAT

The protein derived from animal sources is very acidic to the human body and it causes acids to rise in the blood stream. It's been shown over and over again that excess proteins and acids stress kidneys, too. High protein and fat consumption can contribute to cancer, heart disease, arthritis, kidney and liver problems, and osteoporosis.

Protein isn't just in meat. It can be found in all natural foods -- vegetables and fruits have protein as have nuts, seeds (especially hemp seeds), which can satisfy even the higher protein demands of pregnant women, athletes, and people trying to gain lean muscle mass.

WHAT FOODS CAN I PUT INTO MY RAW VEGAN RECIPES?

Using raw vegan recipes to prepare your food is a great way to live a healthy life. But there are many limitations to what you can use. You can't use any meat. You also can't use any products that come from animals. So that means no milk, no cheese, and no eggs. Oh, and now you've decided that you aren't going to allow yourself too cook anything. So what is there left to eat? Many people avoid using raw vegan recipes because they don't think that there can be any variety. But you would be surprised how many things that you can include in your meals.

The typical diet does not contain a lot of fruits and vegetables, even though it should. When the average person does happen to sneak a fruit into their daily routine it is usually something common like an apple, or a banana. If you are going to be making raw vegan recipes, you have to stretch your mind far beyond your average fruits. There are hundreds of different fruits that you can buy. A lot of people who use this diet will even grow their own food. This opens up a whole bunch of possibilities.

You can also combine those fruits in vegetables into an endless number of combinations when you make smoothies. This can be a fun, entertaining, and delicious way to start your day. I wonder what kiwi, peaches, grapes, and melon would taste like all blended up? You can even add extra flare with different herbs and spices like mint.

You can also find raw vegan recipes that will include nuts, seeds, grains, and legumes. In fact, some people will subscribe to one specific food group. Sproutarians, fruitarians, and juice arians restrict themselves more by adhering to one particular group. But restrictions create possibilities in the raw vegan world. You just have to be creative in your combinations, and preparation.

Don't be scared away from a raw food diet because of its limitations. There are more possibilities out there that you are probably not aware of. If you are committed to living this lifestyle do some research so you can have some fun and colorful meals every day. Raw veganism might be about simplifying life, but it does not have to make life boring.

CHAPTER 2

EASY AND HEALTHY VEGAN BREAKFAST RECIPES

SOUTHWEST SCRAMBLE WITH GREENS (TOFU)

Ingredients

- 1 tbsp. olive oil
- 6 small red potatoes, quartered
- 4 scallions, chopped
- ¼ red onion, minced
- 1 red bell pepper, chopped
- 1 green bell pepper, chopped
- 1 block extra-firm tofu, drained
- 1 tbsp. nutritional yeast
- ½ tsp. oregano
- ½ tsp. ground coriander
- ½ tsp. ground cumin
- ½ tsp. black salt
- ½ tsp. turmeric
- ½ tsp. garlic powder

- ¼ cup water
- 1 large or 2 small plum tomatoes, diced
- 2 tbsp. fresh cilantro, chopped
- 4-6 cups kale or turnip greens
- Kosher salt and black pepper to taste
- 1 garlic clove, minced
- 1/8 tsp. ground nutmeg
- 1 avocado, peeled and sliced
- Juice of ½ lime

Preparation

1. Put the quartered potatoes in a small pot and cover them with cool water. Cover and parboil the potatoes, about 5-7 minutes. Alternatively, you could place the potatoes in a bowl and microwave them for 4-5 minutes on high.
2. Heat the oil in a large sauté pan on medium high. Transfer the parboiled potatoes into the sauté pan and cook until browned, turning them halfway through. When the potatoes are browned, add the scallions, onions, and peppers to the pan and cook, stirring, until softened and tender, about 5 minutes. Crumble tofu into pan and let it cook until slightly browned, about 5 minutes.
3. While the tofu is cooking, prepare the spice mixture. Add the spices to the pan, mixing it well into the tofu and vegetables. The tofu should be yellow from the turmeric. Add the water to the pan and mix. The water helps

incorporate the spices throughout the scramble and moistens the tofu. Turn off the heat. Add the tomatoes to the scramble and mix in the cilantro. Transfer the tofu scramble to a bowl.
4. Prepare the greens in the same pan. If the pan is dry, you can add a bit more oil. Over medium heat, add the greens, garlic, salt, pepper, and nutmeg. Mix well and add a few spoons of water. Cover the pan and cook until just wilted and bright green. Remove from the heat.
5. Arrange a layer of greens on the plates. Layer the tofu scramble on top of the greens.
6. Top with the sliced avocado and lime juice. Enjoy!

PROTEIN OAT BOWL

Ingredients

- Oats
- 1 c plus 2-3 TBSP non-dairy milk of choice
- 1 scoop chocolate vegan protein powder of your choice
- 1 TBSP organic chia seeds
- 1/3 oats, gluten free
- 1-2 TBSP peanut butter
- 1/2- 1 banana, sliced
- 1 TBSP sweet cacao nibs, optional

Instructions

In a container mix together oats, chia seeds, and 1 cup of milk, cover and refrigerator overnight. In the morning add the chocolate protein and additional milk as needed to desired consistency, I usually add about 2 tablespoons. Top with peanut butter, sliced bananas, and optional cacao nibs.

BREAKFAST BURRITOS

Ingredients

- 2 lbs. mixed baby potatoes, cubed
- drizzle of olive oil
- sprinkling of seasoning salt
- dash of ground black pepper
- 1 Tbsp. olive oil
- 3 garlic cloves, minced
- 1 lb. firm tofu, drained and pressed
- 2 tsp. ground cumin
- 1 tsp. dried thyme
- 1 tsp. kosher salt
- ½ tsp. ground turmeric
- 2 Tbsp. water
- heaping ¼ cup nutritional yeast
- 6 frozen vegan breakfast burrito patties, thawed
- 6 burrito sized flour tortillas
- dollop of vegan mayonnaise
- 8 oz. package of vegan shredded cheese
- dollop of salsa

- sprinkling of cilantro, chopped

Preparation

1. First, remove the breakfast patties so they can thaw out.

2. Preheat the oven to 400 F.

3. Wash, dry, and cube the potatoes. Spread them evenly on a rimmed baking sheet and coat with a drizzle of olive oil. Sprinkle with a seasoning salt and a dash of ground black pepper. Stir well to coat evenly and bake at 400 F for about 40 minutes, until fork tender.

4. In a large rimmed frying pan, heat 1 Tbsp. olive oil over medium-low. Add the minced garlic and sauté for a few minutes until fragrant.

5. Next, coat the pan with a nonstick cooking spray and crumble in the tofu with your hands. Sauté for about 5 minutes over medium heat.

6. Meanwhile, whisk together the cumin through and including the water in a small bowl. Add to the tofu and continue to cook for another 10 minutes, scraping up bits that stick to the pan with a metal spatula.

7. Then, stir in the nutritional yeast.

8. Once the tofu is done, transfer to a serving bowl.

9. Add the breakfast patties to the frying pan and break apart into small pieces with a metal spatula. Cook over medium heat for about 5-8 minutes, until browned.

10. Add the tofu back to the pan to warm and combine if you like.

11. Warm the tortillas in the microwave for about 30 seconds.

12. To assemble, place a dollop of mayo in the middle of the tortilla, followed by a pile of potatoes, then some breakfast patty and tofu scramble, a bit of cheese, followed by salsa and cilantro. Fold in the left and right sides first, and then roll away from you to form a burrito!Serve warm with additional salsa if you like.

CREAMY PUMPKIN ACAI BOWL

Ingredients

- 1/2 avocado
- 1 cup vegan milk, such as almond milk or coconut milk, etc.
- 2 tablespoon acai

- 1 tablespoon lucuma powder or 1/2 banana (or both if you like it sweeter)
- 1 pinch cinnamon
- Toppings
- roasted pumpkin
- fresh tahini
- cacao nibs
- raw pistachios
- mulberries for a touch of extra sweetness.

Preparation

1. Blend everything in your high-speed blender (except toppings)
2. Top up with the above toppings or the one of your choice.

MAPLE GINGER PANCAKES

Ingredients

- 1 cup flour
- 1 Tbsp. baking powder
- 1/2 tsp. kosher salt
- 1/4 tsp. ground ginger
- 1/4 tsp. pumpkin pie spice
- 1/3 cup maple syrup
- 3/4 cup water

- 1/4 cup + 1 Tbsp. crystallized ginger slices, minced (plus a little extra for garnish)

Preparation

1. In a medium bowl whisk together the first five ingredients.

2. Make a little hole within the flour mixture and add in the syrup and the water. Stir a few times gently, then add in the chopped ginger and stir until just combined. There might be sprays of flour and that's okay. Do not overmix.

3. Over low, heat a large frying pan. Coat with a nonstick cooking spray. Once the pan is heated, pour in 1/4 cup of the batter. Allow to cook until it starts to form bubbles, then coat the top of the pancake with the nonstick cooking spray and flip. Allow to cook until browned and cooked through.

4. Repeat with the remainder of the batter. This will make about seven medium pancakes.

5. Serve warm and topped with a slathering of vegan butter, a splash of maple syrup and garnished with chopped candied ginger.

CHOCOLATE CHIP, APRICOT, AND ORANGE SCONES

Ingredients

- 2 1/2 cups white whole wheat flour
- 4 tsp. baking powder
- 1/2 tsp. salt
- zest from one orange
- 1 tbsp. egg replacer + 3 tbsp. water (whisk until frothy, then set aside for a minute or two)
- 1/4 cup vegan butter
- 4 oz. unsweetened applesauce
- 1/4 cup pure maple syrup
- 1/4-1/2 cup soy milk
- 1/2 cup vegan chocolate chips or chocolate chunks
- 1/2 cup dried apricots, chopped
- ~2 tbsp. soy milk, for brushing tops of scones
- Demerara sugar, for sprinkling, if desired

Preparation

1. Line a baking sheet with parchment paper and preheat the oven to 425F.

2. In a large bowl, whisk together the flour, baking soda, salt and orange zest. Add the butter in chunks and blend until the mixture is the consistency of coarse meal.

3. In a small bowl, whisk together the egg replacer, applesauce, maple syrup and soy milk, then pour into the dry ingredients – adding more soy milk if necessary. Just before the dough is thoroughly combined, stir in the chocolate chips and dried apricots.

4. Scoop the batter into a ball and place on a floured surface (or directly onto the lined baking pan). Pat dough into a circle that is about 1/2" thick. Move the circle onto the baking sheet and cut into 8-12 pieces. Separate the triangles a little bit, then brush the tops with soy milk and sprinkle with sugar.

5. Bake for 15-20 minutes or until tops are a nice, rich brown. Let the scones cool for a minute before putting on wire cooling racks. Eat while still warm!

CINNAMON APPLE 'TOAST'

Ingredients

- 1 cup walnuts, soaked overnight
- 5 dates, soaked for ~15 minutes
- 1 apple, cored
- 1 small sweet potato, peeled and cut into small pieces (about 1 cup)
- 1/2 cup unsweetened apple juice
- 1/2 of a banana
- 1 1/2 tsp. cinnamon
- 1/4 tsp. cardamom

- pinch salt, optional
- 1 cup flaxseed meal
- 1/4 cup flaxseeds
- 1/4 cup raw sunflower seeds
- 1/4 cup raw hulled hemp seeds

Preparation

1. In a food processor, process the walnuts through the salt until nearly smooth. You'll need to scrape down the bowl of the processor a few times.

2. In a large bowl, combine the flaxseed meal, flaxseeds, sunflower seeds, and hemp seeds. Pour in the walnut mixture and stir until thoroughly combined. Spread the mixture onto a Teflex dehydrator sheet to just a hair under 1/2" thick and neaten up the edges. Gently score the dough into desired shapes. Place in the dehydrator and dehydrate at 145F for 30 minutes, then turn down the temperature to 115F and continue to dehydrate the "toast" until is dry and very crispy, about 20-24 hours.

3. Tip: about 2 hours in, carefully flip the "toast" by placing a mesh sheet + dehydrator tray on top of it, and then, gently remove the Teflex sheet. This speeds up the dehydrating process.

4. Break the "toast" into pieces and store in an air-tight container. To serve, top with fruit-sweetened jam, natural almond or peanut butter – or your favorite toast toppings. 5. For crackers, spread the batter to about 1/4" – you'll need two trays and the drying time will be less.

POMEGRANATE QUINOA PORRIDGE

Ingredients

- 1 1/2 cup quinoa flakes
- 3 cups milk almond milk
- 2 1/2 teaspoons cinnamon (add more if needed)
- 1 teaspoon vanilla extract
- 10 organic prunes, pitted and cut into 1/4's
- 1 pomegranate pulp
- 1/4 cup desiccated coconut
- stewed apples (2 apples granny smith, 1/2 cup purified water)
- coconut flakes to garnish

Preparation

1. Place quinoa and almond milk into saucepan, and stir on medium to low heat for

2. approximately 7 minutes, until smooth consistency

3. Add cinnamon, desiccated coconut and vanilla extract (add more if needed) and taste

4. Pit prunes and cut into quarters, add to porridge stir in well

5. Serve into individual bowls

6. Add scoop of stewed apple (see recipe below), pomegranates (use the juice from pomegranate), prunes and coconut flakes

7. Ready to eat!

STEWED APPLES

1. Peel, core, slice apples and place into saucepan with water
2. Cook apples on a medium heat, until soft
3. Remove from heat, drain and mash apples
4. Ready to serve!

MEXICAN-SPICED TOFU SCRAMBLE

Ingredients

- 2 packages of extra-firm tofu, drained, and pressed
- 1 tbsp. safflower oil
- 3 scallions, chopped

- 1 red bell pepper, chopped
- 2 cloves garlic, minced
- ½ tsp. ground cumin
- ½ tsp. ground coriander
- ½ tsp. Mexican chile powder
- ½ tsp. paprika
- ½ tsp. dried oregano
- ½ tsp. garlic powder
- 1 tsp. black salt
- 1/2 tsp. turmeric
- 2 tbsp. nutritional yeast (optional)
- 2 tbsp. ground flaxseed (optional)
- 1 cup water
- 1-4 oz. can green chiles
- 1-15 oz. can black beans, drained and rinsed
- 2 tbsp. fresh cilantro, chopped

Preparation

1. Heat a large, deep skillet over medium heat. Add the oil, then cook the scallions, bell pepper and garlic for about 3 minutes until softened. Break the tofu into large chunks and add to the pan. Toss it, so it's covered with the aromatics and then let it sit so it browns a little before flipping it.

When it browns after about 5 minutes, toss the tofu to let it brown on all sides.

2. While the tofu is browning, make the spice mix in a small bowl or cup. Increase or decrease the amounts based on how spicy you like your food. Nutritional yeast and flaxseed are optional, but healthy additions if you have them. Add the spice mix to the pan and toss the tofu to distribute the spices evenly. Add 1 cup of water to the pan and stir. This helps the spices distribute evenly and moistens the scramble. The water will cook out.

3. Mix the green chiles and the black beans into the tofu scramble. Let cook about 5 minutes until all the ingredients are heated through. Stir in the cilantro. Serve while hot.

CHEWY HOMEMADE GRANOLA BARS (GLUTEN FREE)

Ingredients

- 1 – 2 tsp. coconut oil, for greasing pan or cooking spray
- ½ cup cashews, raw & unsalted
- 4 cups Gluten Free Extra Thick Rolled Oats
- ½ cup dried cranberries
- ½ tsp. cinnamon
- ½ cup semi-sweet chocolate chips (soy, dairy & gluten free)
- 3 Tbsp. flaxseed meal
- 1 cup peanut butter

- 1/3 cup brown rice syrup
- ½ cup brown sugar
- 1 vanilla bean or 1 tsp. pure vanilla extract
- 1 ripe banana, mashed

Preparation

1. Preheat oven to 350 degrees F.

2. Spread raw cashews on a baking sheet and bake for 8 minutes. Allow to cool.

3. Meanwhile lightly grease a square brownie pan or 9×13 inch pan with coconut oil; alternatively you can use cooking spray.

4. When the cashews are cooled, chop them into smaller pieces.

5. In a large mixing bowl combine the dry ingredients – cashew pieces, oats, cranberries, cinnamon, chocolate chips, and flaxseed meal, stir and set aside.

6. Using a paring knife, carefully slice the vanilla bean in half lengthwise. Using the back of the knife, gently run it along the inside of the vanilla bean scraping the seeds out. Repeat

for the other half of the vanilla bean. Alternatively you can use 1 tsp. pure vanilla extract.

7. In a medium saucepan over low heat add vanilla bean seeds, peanut butter, brown rice syrup, brown sugar, and mashed banana. Stir for a few minutes until melted and mixed together.

8. Add the peanut butter syrup mixture to the large mixing bowl with oats. Stir until everything is evenly coated.

9. Place granola into the pan. Press down firmly with the back of a spoon or the back of a measuring cup.

10. Refrigerate granola for 50 minutes and then freeze for 10 minutes before removing from pan and/or cutting.

11. Keep granola bars stored in the fridge in an airtight container for up to 1 week.

CHAPTER 3

EASY AND HEALTHY VEGAN LUNCH RECIPES

MEXICAN AVOCADO SALAD

Ingredients:

- 24 cherry tomatoes, quartered
- 1 tablespoon extra-virgin olive oil
- 2 teaspoons red wine vinegar
- 1 teaspoon salt
- ¼ teaspoon freshly ground black pepper
- ½ medium yellow or white onion, finely chopped
- 1 jalapeño, seeded and finely chopped
- 2 tablespoons chopped fresh cilantro
- ¼ medium head iceberg lettuce, cut into ½-inch ribbons
- 2 ripe Hass avocados, seeded, peeled, and chopped

Directions:

1. Combine tomatoes, oil, vinegar, salt, and pepper in a medium bowl; let them stand at room temperature for 1 hour. Add onion, jalapeño and cilantro; toss well.
2. Arrange lettuce on a platter and top with avocado. Spoon tomato mixture on top and serve.

CRAZY DELICIOUS RAW PAD THAI

Ingredients

- 2 large zucchini
- ¼ red cabbage, thinly sliced
- ¼ cup fresh mint leaves, chopped
- 1 spring onion, sliced
- ½ avocado, peeled, and sliced
- 12 raw almonds
- 2 tbsp sesame seeds

Dressing

- ¼ cup peanut butter (100% natural with no added salt or sugar)
- 1 tbsp tahini
- 1 lemon, juiced
- 2 tbsp tamari / salt-reduced soy sauce
- ½ chopped green chili (or more if you like the hot stuff!)

Preparation

1. Assemble dressing ingredients in a jar. Pop the lid on and shake well to combine. I like mine nice and creamy, but you can add a touch of filtered water if it looks too thick.

2. Using a mandoline or vegetable peeler, remove one outer strip of skin from each zucchini and discard. Peel again, in long strips and periodically rotating the zucchini, to create 'ribbons' from all around the core. Discard the core or use it in another recipe (or juice it!).

3. Combine zucchini ribbons, cabbage and dressing in a large mixing bowl and mix well.

4. Divide zucchini mixture between two plates or bowls.

5. Top with remaining ingredients and enjoy!

KALE & WILD RICE STIR FLY

Ingredients

- 1 tsp extra virgin olive oil or coconut oil
- ¼ onion, diced
- 3 carrots, cut into ½ inch slices
- 2 cups assorted mushrooms
- 1 bunch kale, chopped into bite sized pieces
- 1 tbsp lemon juice
- 1 tsp chili flakes, more if desired
- 1 tablespoon Braggs Liquid Aminos or Braggs Soy
- 1 cup wild rice, cooked

Instructions

1. In a large sauté pan, heat oil over medium heat. Add in onion and cook until translucent, about 3-5 minutes.
2. Add in carrots and sauté another 3 minutes. Add in mushrooms and cook 2 minutes. Add in kale, lemon juice, chili flakes, and Braggs. Cook until kale is slightly wilted.
3. Serve over wild rice.
4. Extra tip: Can top with fresh chopped avocado and red pepper flakes

EXTRA CREAMY MAC AND CHEESE

Ingredients

- 1 russet potato, peeled and cut into bite-sized pieces (1 1/2 cups/ 240g)
- 1 cup carrot, cut into 1/2 inch rounds (130g)
- 1/4 yellow onion, diced (1/2 cup/ 65g)
- 2 cups water (470ml)
- 1/2 cup Earth Balance spread (72g)
- 1/2 cup nutritional yeast (40g)
- 1/2 teaspoon turmeric
- 1 teaspoon salt (6g)
- 3 tablespoons coconut milk (45ml)
- 3 turns fresh black pepper
- 1 box (8 oz. / 227g) gluten free pasta (Garden Pagodas quinoa pasta by Ancient

Harvest is my fave), or regular elbows.

- Parsley for garnish

Preparation

Cheese Sauce

1. Place potato, carrot and onion in a pan, cover with 2 cups of water and simmer for 20 minutes with the lid on.

2. After 20 minutes, turn off heat and add Earth Balance spread, nutritional yeast, turmeric, and salt. Stir to combine until melted.

3. Pour mixture into a blender and blend until creamy and smooth, about a minute on medium. You may need to scrape the sides down from the blender a couple of times for everything to get incorporated.

4. Add coconut milk to the blender and continue to blend until mixture is creamy throughout.

5. Leave in the blender for now.

Pasta

1. Cook pasta according to the directions on the box.

2. Strain pasta and rinse with cold water to stop from cooking. Return to pan.
3. Turn heat on very low and pour cheese sauce over pasta.
4. Add black pepper and stir to combine.
5. Turn off heat and serve.
6. Garnish with parsley.

GRILLED BUFFALO TOFU PO' BOY WITH APPLE SLAW

Ingredients

- ½ cup vegetable broth
- ¼ cup hot sauce, plus more for serving
- 1 tablespoon vegan butter
- 1 (14 to 16-ounces) package tofu, pressed overnight, and cut into ½-inch slices
- 4 cups shredded cabbage
- 2 medium apples, grated
- 1 medium shallot, grated
- 6 tablespoons vegan mayonnaise, plus more for spreading
- 1 tablespoon apple cider vinegar
- Salt and black pepper
- 4 (6-inch) hoagie rolls or gluten-free wraps
- 8 slices tomato

Preparation

1. Combine the broth, hot sauce and butter in a medium saucepan. Bring the sauce to a boil, add the tofu slices and reduce to a simmer. Simmer the tofu for 10 minutes. Remove the pan from the heat and set aside for 10 minutes to marinate.
2. Combine the cabbage, apple, shallot, mayo and vinegar in a large bowl. Season with salt and black pepper and mix well.
3. Heat a large grill pan over medium heat. Drain the tofu, reserving the marinade. Grill the tofu until heated through and grill marks appear, about 5 minutes per side. Baste the tofu with the reserved marinade, as needed.
4. Toast the hoagie rolls or warm the wraps. To assemble the sandwiches, spread a few teaspoons of mayo on the rolls or wraps. Add 2 slices of tomato and two slices of grilled tofu to each sandwich. Top with more hot sauce, if desired, and add slaw, to taste. Serve.

MEXICAN BLACK BEAN SOUP

Ingredients

- 2 tbsp extra virgin olive oil
- 1 onion, diced
- 3 cloves garlic, minced
- 2 carrots, diced
- 2 celery stalks, diced
- 1 red bell pepper, diced

- 1 green bell pepper, diced
- 1 cup organic corn
- 1 can black beans
- 2 Tbsp chili powder
- ½ Tbsp paprika
- ½ Tbsp crushed red pepper flakes
- ½ Tbsp dried oregano
- ½ Tbsp black pepper
- Himalayan rock salt, to taste
- 4 cups vegetable broth
- 2 Tbsp nutritional yeast
- 1 lime juiced
- 1 avocado, diced
- Cilantro for a garnish
- Organic corn chips *optional

Preparation

1. Heat olive oil in a large pot at medium heat. Sauté onions until translucent, roughly 5 minutes.
2. Add garlic, carrots, celery, peppers and corn and sauté until soft, roughly 5 minutes.
3. Add black beans, spices, salt to taste and veggie broth. Bring to a boil and then lower and simmer for 20 to 30 minutes. Finally stir in the nutritional yeast and lime juice.
4. Serve hot topped with cilantro, avocado and crumbled organic corn chips.

CRAB CAKES WITH SWEET BALSAMIC MAYO

Ingredients

- 3 cups cooked Garbanzo beans (see note if you want to pressure cook your own)
- 1 1/2 cup gluten free crackers, ground up (I used Sesmark Gluten Free Rice Thins)
- 2 green onions, finely chopped (use entire onion)
- 1/2 cup red bell pepper, diced
- 3 tablespoons red onion, diced
- 2 tablespoons fresh parsley, chopped
- 1 teaspoon Wasabi mustard
- 1 tablespoon fresh lemon juice
- 1/4 cup ground flax seeds
- 1 teaspoon garlic powder
- 1 teaspoon dulse flakes or powder
- 1 teaspoon salt
- 10 turns freshly ground Black pepper
- 1/2 cup Grapeseed oil

Preparation

1. Place the crackers in a food processor and process until they are ground up, resembling flour. Measure out 1/3 of a cup and set aside (if you end up with more than 1/3 of a cup, store the remainder in a container for another time).
2. Place the garbanzo beans in the food processor and pulse several times until the beans are processed but not smooth

like paste. Even if you have a few whole beans, that is okay.
3. In a large bowl, place the garbanzo beans, processed crackers, green onions, red bell pepper, red onion, parsley, mustard, lemon juice, ground flax seeds, garlic powder, dulse, salt and black pepper.
4. Stir ingredients together. The mixture will be on the dry side, this is a good sign. If it's easier, mix everything with your hands.
5. Form the mixture into 6 equal patties. Make them fat and round (you will be pressing them out a little in the next step).
6. Heat the oil in a large enough pan to hold all 6 (if you do not have a large enough pan,
7. you will need to fry them in two batches).
8. When the oil is hot (I mean hot, not warm. To test if the oil is hot enough, put a small amount of water on your fingertips and flick the water in the oil. If it sizzles, you're ready to go).
9. Place the Crab Cakes in the oil and allow to cook until the underside gets brown, about 5 minutes. Flip and cook until crab cake is brown on the other side.
10. Make the mayo below and serve on your favorite gluten free bread / bun. Alternatively, you can serve this on top of mixed greens and topped with the mayo.

CRISPY TOFU NUGGETS

Ingredients

For the Tofu Nuggets

- ½ cup all-purpose flour (65 g)
- 1 teaspoon raw cane sugar
- 1 teaspoon sea salt
- 2¾ cups unsweetened cornflakes (100 g)
- 14 ounces tofu (400 g)
- 2 cups vegetable oil (500 mL)

For the Curry Ketchup

- Juice from ½ lemon
- ⅔ cup tomato paste (140 g)
- 2 tablespoons agave syrup
- 1 teaspoon curry powder
- 2 tablespoons olive oil
- Sea salt
- Freshly ground black pepper

Preparation

For the Tofu Nuggets

1. Stir the flour together with the raw cane sugar, sea salt, and 6 tablespoons (90 mL) water until the batter is smooth.

2. Finely crumble the cornflakes.

3. Cut the tofu into slices that are just under ½ inch (1 cm), and then use a knife to shape the tofu into nuggets.

4. Dip the nuggets in the batter and then coat them with the cornflakes.

5. Heat the vegetable oil in a deep fryer or a small saucepan. (You'll know the oil is hot enough if you dip a wooden toothpick into the oil and small bubbles float up to the top around the toothpick.)

6. Fry the nuggets for approx. 3 minutes.

7. Transfer to a plate lined with paper towels to absorb any excess oil.

For the Curry Ketchup

1. Mix all of the ingredients with 3 tablespoons water.
2. Serve with the nuggets.

BLACK BEAN VEGAN WRAPS

Ingredients

- 1 1/2 half cup of beans (sprouted and cooked)
- 1 carrot
- 2 tomatoes
- 1 avocado
- One cob of corn
- kale
- two or three sticks of celery
- 2 persimmons
- coriander
- Dressing:
- 1 hachiya persimmon (or half a mango)
- Juice of 1 lemon
- 3 tablespoons olive oil
- 1/4 cup water
- 1 teaspoon grated fresh ginger
- 1/2 teaspoon of salt

Preparation

1. Sprout and cook the black beans.
2. Chop the ingredients and mix them in a bowl with the black beans.
3. Blend the ingredients for the dressing and pour into the salad. Serve a spoonful in a lettuce leaf that you can quickly roll into a wrap. I recommend iceberg or romaine lettuce.

SOUTHWESTERN VEGAN GRILLED CHEESE SANDWICH

Ingredients

- 1 small sweet potato, sliced thinly
- 1/2 cup sweet bell peppers, sliced
- 1 cup beans – Kidney or Black
- 1/2 cup salsa
- 4 slices bread
- 1 – 2 tablespoons dairy-free margarine
- Vegan Jalapeño Garlic Havarti Wedge

Preparation

1. Coat a skillet with vegetable spray and cook the sweet potatoes and sweet bell peppers over medium heat until tender. This usually takes 5 – 10 minutes at most. That's one thing I love about sweet potatoes, they're just ready to be cooked! Place the potatoes and peppers on a plate and set aside to cool.

2. In a bowl, combine the beans and the salsa and mash with a fork. You can follow your preference as to whether you mash the beans into a paste (like refried beans) or leave it with some of the beans whole.

3. Place the same skillet you used for the sweet potatoes over medium heat. While you're waiting for the skillet to warm up, slather margarine onto one side of each slice of bread. Place two slices of bread with buttered side down in the skillet. Top with one or two thin slices of Daiya cheese, grilled sweet potatoes, mashed beans, and then one or two thin slices of cheese. Top that with the second piece of prepared bread, this time the buttered side up.

4. Let the bread cook until toasted to your preference. I like to lift up the bottom corner every now and then to make sure it's toasted just right. Once the bottom bread is toasted just so, use a spatula to turn the sandwich (carefully…so you don't lose any good filling) and toast the other side of the sandwich.

5. As the bread is toasting, the heat should also melt the cheese. If not, you can place the sandwich in the microwave and heat for a few seconds at a time until you get everything just right.

CHAPTER 4

EASY AND HEALTHY VEGAN DINNER RECIPES

COUNTRY 'MEATLOAF' WITH GRAVY

Ingredients

Country 'Meatloaf'

- 3 tbsp. olive oil
- 1 large onion, diced
- 2 large carrots, diced
- 2 cups celery, diced
- 8 cloves garlic, minced
- 2 tsp. dried thyme
- 2 tsp. dried basil
- 2 tsp. dried parsley
- 2 (8 oz.) packages tempeh
- 1/2 cup soy sauce or Braggs
- 1/2 cup vegetable broth
- 1 cup cooked brown rice, warm
- 1/2 cup bread crumbs
- Sea salt and freshly ground black pepper

Golden Gravy

- 2 tbsp. canola oil
- 1 large onion, roughly chopped
- 1/4 cup nutritional yeast flakes
- 1/2 cup flour
- 2 cups water
- 3 tbsp. soy sauce
- 1 tsp. dried thyme
- 1 tsp. garlic powder
- Sea salt and freshly ground black pepper

Preparation

1. Preheat oven to 350°F. Lightly grease a 10x5x3 inch loaf pan.

2. Heat oil over medium-high heat in a large deep-sided skillet or dutch oven and sauté onion, carrots, and celery until soft, about 15 minutes. Stir in garlic, thyme, basil and parsley. Let cook a few more minutes. Crumble the tempeh into the skillet and add soy sauce and broth. Reduce heat to medium and cook for about 5 minutes, stirring often. Transfer the mixture to a large bowl.

3. Add warm brown rice and breadcrumbs to the bowl and mix thoroughly with a large spoon. The more you mix it

and mash it, the better it will hold together when you bake it. Season with salt and pepper.

4. Transfer the mixture into the prepared loaf pan and pack it down very firmly using the back of a spoon. Cover the top of the pan with foil. Bake for 45 minutes, covered, then remove foil, and bake for an additional 15 to 20 minutes. Remove from oven and let rest for 5 minutes before unmolding. Run a knife around the edges of the cooked loaf to loosen, then flip onto a serving plate to unmold. Slice and serve.

5. For the gravy: In a medium saucepan, heat oil over medium-high heat and sauté onion until soft. Add nutritional yeast and flour, and stir for about 1 minute. Add water, soy sauce, thyme and garlic powder. Continue to cook, whisking continuously, until mixture is very thick. Transfer gravy to a blender and purée until smooth. Adjust seasonings, and add salt and pepper to taste.

Notes

Recipe can be halved to serve 3 to 4 people. If halving, bake in an 8-by-4-by-3-inch loaf pan for 30 minutes covered, then 15 more minutes uncovered.

ZUCCHINI PASTA WITH PESTO SAUCE

Ingredients

- 2 medium zucchini (make noodles with a mandoline or Spiralizer)
- 1/2 teaspoon salt

For Pesto

- 1/4 cup cashews (soaked)
- 1/4 cup pine nuts (soaked)
- 1/2 cup spinach
- 1/2 cup peas (fresh or frozen)
- 1/4 cup broccoli
- 1/4 cup basil leaves
- 1/2 avocado
- 2 tablespoons olive oil

- 2 tablespoons nutritional yeast

- 1/2 teaspoon salt

- Pinch black pepper

- 1/2 cup water

Preparation

1. Place zucchini noodles in a strainer over a bowl. Add 1/2 teaspoon of salt and let it set while preparing the pesto sauce.

2. Blend all the ingredients for the pesto sauce.

3. Drain excess water from zucchini noodles and place them in a bowl or plate.

4. Pour the sauce on top and garnish with some basil leaves and pine nuts.

TEMPEH FISH N CHIPS W/ TARTAR SAUCE

Ingredients

For the Tempeh "Fish"

- 2 packages of tempeh
- 2 cups chickpea flour
- 1 Tbs. baking powder
- 1 Tbs. garlic powder
- 1 Tbs. chile powder
- 2 tsp. Old Bay seasoning
- ¼ cup cider vinegar
- 12 oz. seltzer
- 1 cup corn starch
- 1 Tbs. kelp flakes
- Safflower oil for frying

For the Chips

- 4 large russet potatoes cut into wedges
- Cooking oil spray
- Salt and pepper to taste
- ½ tsp. garlic powder
- ½ tsp. paprika

For the Tartar Sauce

- 1 cup Vegan mayonnaise
- 2 Tbs. unsweetened pickle relish
- 1 tsp. lemon zest
- Juice of half a lemon

Instructions

For the Tempeh "Fish"

1. Split the tempeh in half so that you have two thin rectangles. The way I do this is to lay the tempeh on a cutting board, hold the top steady with the palm of your hand and with a knife, slice through it like you are splitting open a bagel.

2. If you like your tempeh less chewy, steam it for a few minutes to soften it. Cut each piece of tempeh into 4 pieces so you will have 16 pieces in total.

3. In a bowl, add the flour, baking powder, garlic powder, chile powder, and Old Bay seasoning. Mix well. Add in the vinegar and slowly mix in the seltzer until the batter is the desired consistency (like pancake batter). In another bowl, mix the corn starch and the kelp flakes.

4. Heat 2 inches of oil in a large skillet. Dredge the tempeh pieces into the corn starchkelp mixture, shake off the excess, and then coat with the batter. If you want an extra

crunchy, thicker battered covering, re-dredge the tempeh a second time. Fry the tempeh in the skillet in batches, turning once, until golden brown. Place the pieces on paper towels to drain and sprinkle with salt.

5. Serve while hot with chips and tartar sauce on the side. Add lemon wedges for garnish, if desired.

For the Chips

1. Preheat oven to 425°F with a baking sheet in the oven.

2. Pull the hot sheet pan out of the oven and put potato wedges on it in a single layer.

3. Spray with cooking spray, sprinkle the spices onto the potatoes and put them back into the oven.

4. Bake the potatoes, turning occasionally, until golden brown and tender, about 40 minutes. For the Tartar Sauce

1. In a bowl, mix the Vegan mayonnaise with the unsweetened pickle relish. Add some lemon zest and the juice of half a lemon. Mix well.

2. Refrigerate until ready to serve.

VEGAN MUSHROOM STROGANOFF

Ingredients

- 8 oz. uncooked ribbon noodles (230g)
- 1 tablespoon olive oil (15ml)
- 1 yellow onion, chopped (140g)
- 3 tablespoons whole wheat flour, divided (20g)
- 2 cups beefless beef broth or veggie broth (0.5 liters) 1 tablespoon soy sauce (15ml)
- 1 teaspoon lemon juice (5ml) 1 teaspoon tomato paste (6g)
- 1 1/2 pounds mushrooms (half portobello and half button mushrooms), cut into large
- 2-inch chunks (740g)
- 1/2 teaspoon dried thyme 1/2 teaspoon dried sage 1/2 teaspoon salt (3g)
- 1 tablespoon white wine vinegar (15ml) 1/4 cup vegan sour cream – optional (55g) 10 turns of fresh ground, black pepper 1/4 cup flat-leaf parsley, minced (6g)

Instructions

1. Cook the noodles per the direction on the package. Undercook them a bit because they will be cooked again once incorporated into the sauce.
2. Drain, and set aside.
3. In a large saucepan, add the olive oil and sauté the onions for three minutes on medium heat.
4. Add the flour and cook for 30 seconds, stirring constantly.

5. Gradually add the broth, soy sauce, lemon juice and tomato paste, while stirring at the same time. Stir until mixture becomes thick and bubbly, about a minute.
6. Add the mushrooms, thyme, sage and salt. Stir to combine.
7. Cook for 5 minutes, stirring frequently until mushrooms have shrunk in size.
8. Add the vinegar and simmer for 4 more minutes.
9. Add the noodles, sour cream, 1 tablespoon of flour, black pepper and parsley and cook on low for an additional 5 minutes.
10. Garnish with parsley.

THE VEGAN EGGPLANT CRUNCHBURGER

Ingredients

For the Horseradish Mustard Mayo

- 1/4 cup vegan mayonnaise
- 2 Tbs. Dijon mustard
- 2 Tbs. prepared horseradish
- A pinch of dried tarragon
- Kosher salt and black pepper to taste

For the eggplant burgers

- 1 large or 2 medium eggplants, peeled and cubed
- 2 Tbs. extra-virgin olive oil, divided

- 1 shallot, finely minced
- 1 cup vegan cheese shreds, any flavor
- 1 clove garlic, minced or grated
- ½ tsp. Kosher salt
- ¼ tsp. black pepper
- 1 Tbs. fresh parsley, chopped
- 1 cup gluten-free breadcrumbs

For the toppings

- 1 cup vegan cheese, either slices or shreds (as long as it melts)
- 4 gluten-free buns
- 4 slices beefsteak tomato
- 4 leaves romaine lettuce
- 4 slices red onion
- Horseradish Mustard Mayonnaise (recipe above)
- 4 handfuls of potato chips

Preparation

For the Horseradish Mustard Mayo

1. Whisk together the mayonnaise, mustard, and horseradish in a small bowl and season with salt and pepper.
2. Cover and refrigerate for at least 30 minutes to allow the flavors to meld.

3. The sauce can be prepared 1 day in advance and kept covered in the refrigerator.

To make the Eggplant Burgers

1. In a large skillet, heat 1 Tbs. of the oil over medium-high heat. Add the eggplant cubes and sauté until they are browned and very soft, about 10-12 minutes. Make sure they are super-soft because they need to be mashed. You could also roast the eggplant to make it soft.

2. Transfer the eggplant to a large bowl. Mash the eggplant up until there are no whole pieces left. Use a potato masher to do this. Once you have a big bowl of mush, add the shallot, cheese, garlic, salt, pepper, and parsley. Mix it into the eggplant. Add the bread crumbs. Don't add them all at once; you want to feel the mix and see whether you need a whole cup. I add ½ cup of bread crumbs and mix it.

3. The best way to mix it is wet your hands and use one hand (keep the other hand clean) to gently mix the crumbs into the eggplant. You will probably need more crumbs so add another ¼ cup and mix it again. You want the consistency to feel firm like it will hold up as a burger. If it feels too moist, add the last ¼ cup of bread crumbs. Usually, I end up using the whole cup of crumbs.

4. Put the eggplant mixture into the fridge for about 30 minutes. Take the bowl out of the fridge and with your hand, divide the mixture into 4 parts. To form the burgers, I use a 3 ½ inch cookie cutter. I spray it with a bit of cooking oil spray and then pack the eggplant mixture into the cookie cutter. Pat it down, let it sit for about 20 seconds and then gently lift the cookie cutter off. Let your perfect burger sit for a few minutes undisturbed while you make the other 3 burgers.

5. In the same skillet that you sautéed the eggplant in (but cleaned), heat the other Tbs. of oil over medium-high heat and add the burgers to the pan. Let cook until slightly browned on one side and (this is very important); you can lift the burger with a spatula without breaking it. I use 2 spatulas to gently turn the burgers. Flip them and let them cook on the other side. When the 2nd side gets golden brown, flip them back over and let the first side cook until golden brown.

To make the Vegan Crunchburgers

1. Top the burgers with either 2 slices or ¼ cup of vegan cheese. Add about a Tbs. of water to the pan and cover it. This will create steam and allow the cheese to melt and get ooey-gooey.

2. If you want your buns toasty, put on some pants. If you want your burger buns toasty, preheat the broiler while you

are cooking the burgers. Split the buns and put the halves, cut side up, on a baking sheet and cook them until they are lightly golden brown, about 30 seconds. Don't burn them!!

3. Place the burgers on the bun bottoms and, if desired, top with tomato, lettuce, onion, and a dollop of horseradish mustard mayonnaise. Pile on the potato chips, top with the bun tops, and serve immediately. Make sure you have tons of napkins because it's going to be messy.

BALSAMIC BBQ SEITAN AND TEMPEH RIBS

Ingredients

For the spice rub

- 1/4 cup raw turbinado sugar
- 2 Tbs. smoked paprika
- 1 tsp. cayenne pepper
- 3 garlic cloves, minced
- 2 tsp. dried oregano
- 1 Tbs. Kosher salt
- 1 ½ tsp. ground black pepper
- ¼ cup fresh parsley, minced

For the Balsamic BBQ Sauce

- ½ cup apple cider vinegar
- ¾ cup balsamic vinegar
- ¾ cup maple syrup
- 1 1/2 cups ketchup
- 1 red onion, minced
- 1 garlic clove, minced
- 1 serrano chile, seeded and minced

For the Seitan Ribs

- 2 cups vital wheat gluten
- 3 Tbs. Mexican chile powder
- 3 Tbs. dried onion powder
- 3 Tbs. dried garlic powder
- ¼ cup nutritional yeast
- ½ tsp. ground black pepper
- 2 cups water
- ¼ cup tahini
- ¼ cup low-sodium soy sauce
- 2 tsp. liquid smoke

Preparation

1. In a small bowl, combine the ingredients for the spice rub. Mix well and set aside.

2. In a small saucepan over medium heat, combine the apple cider vinegar, balsamic vinegar, maple syrup, ketchup, red onion, garlic and chile. Stir and let simmer, uncovered, for

about an hour. Increase the heat to medium-high and cook for 15 more minutes until the sauce thickens. Stir it often. If it seems too thick, add some water.

3. Preheat the oven to 350 degrees. In a large bowl, combine the dry ingredients for the seitan and mix well. In a smaller bowl, combine the wet ingredients. Add the wet ingredients to the dry and mix until just combined. Knead the dough lightly until everything is combined and the dough feels elastic.

4. Grease or spray a baking dish. Add the dough to the baking dish, flattening it and stretching it out to fit the dish. Cut the dough into 8 strips and then in half to make 16 thick ribs. (Note: if you want the ribs thin, this is enough dough to fill 2 baking sheets. If you want them thick, it is enough for one).

5. Top the dough with the spice rub and massage it in a bit. Bake the seitan for 40 to 60 minutes or until the seitan has a sturdy texture to it (thinner ribs will cook faster). Remove the dish from the oven. Recut the strips and carefully remove them from the baking dish.

6. Increase the oven temperature to 400 degrees. Slather the ribs with BBQ sauce and lay them on a baking sheet. Put the ribs back in the oven for just about 10 minutes so the sauce can get a bit charred. Alternatively, you can cook the sauce-covered ribs on a grill or in a grill pan.

For the Tempeh Ribs

1. Slice a package of tempeh into 6 or 8 rectangles, depending how wide you want the "ribs" to be. If you want them to be thinner, slice the tempeh in half like a bagel first. Steam the tempeh for 15 minutes until it softens a bit.

2. Coat the tempeh with the spice rub. Cook the tempeh ribs in the oven or in a skillet until browned on both sides. This should take about 8 minutes per side. Brush the BBQ sauce on the tempeh and cook for another few minutes until slightly charred.

GREEN BEAN CASSEROLE

Ingredients

- 1 large onion, diced
- 3 T olive oil
- ¼ c flour
- 2 c water
- 1 tsp salt
- ½ tsp garlic powder
- 2 bags frozen green beans (10 ounces each)
- 1 can fried onions, or make your own

Preparation

1. Preheat oven to 350.

2. Heat olive oil in a shallow pan. Add onion and stir occasionally while the onions soften and turn translucent. This takes a good 20 minutes, don't rush it because it gives so much flavor! Once onion is well cooked, add flour and stir well to cook flour. It will be a dry mixture. Add salt and garlic powder. Add water. Let simmer for a few minutes and allow mixture to thicken. Remove from heat.

3. Pour green beans into a square baking dish and add 2/3 can of onions. Add all of the gravy and stir well to combine. Place in oven and cook for 30 minutes, gravy mixture will be bubbly. Top with remaining fried onions and cook for 5-10 minutes more. Serve immediately!

SOCCA PIZZA [VEGAN]

Ingredients

Socca Base

- 1 cup chickpea (garbanzo bean) flour – I used Bob's Red Mill Garbanzo Fava Flour
- 1 cup cold, filtered water

- 1 tsp minced garlic
- ½ tsp sea salt
- 2 tbsp coconut oil (for greasing)

Toppings

- Tomato paste
- Dried Italian herbs (oregano, basil, thyme, rosemary, etc)
- Mushrooms
- Red onion
- Capsicum/bell pepper
- Sun-dried tomatoes
- Kalamata olives
- Vegan Cheese (Vegusto, etc) – optional

To Serve

- Fresh basil leaves, chopped

Preparation

1. Pre-heat oven to 350F (or slightly higher if your oven is not fan-forced).

2. In a large mixing bowl, whisk together garbanzo bean flour and water until there are no lumps remaining. Stir in garlic and sea salt. Allow to rest for about 10 minutes to thicken slightly.

3. Grease 4 small, shallow dishes/tins with coconut oil.

4. Pour mixture into dishes and bake for about 25 minutes or until golden brown.

5. Remove dishes from oven, top with your favourite toppings and vegan cheese (optional) and return to the oven for another 10 minutes or so.

6. Remove dishes from oven and allow to sit for a few minutes before removing pizzas from the dishes.

7. Top pizzas with fresh basil leaves and enjoy!

SWEET POTATO TOFU PIZZA

Ingredients

- 1 whole wheat pizza crust
- 2 medium sweet potatoes
- 1/4 cup plus 2 tablespoons plain almond milk
- 1 tablespoon vegan butter, softened

- 1 teaspoon sea salt
- 1 teaspoon fresh ground black pepper
- 1/2 cup red onion, diced
- 1 clove of garlic, diced
- 1/2 cup celery, diced
- 1/2 cup yellow bell pepper, diced
- 1 tablespoon coconut oil
- 1/2 block of extra firm tofu, drained and pressed (learn how to make tofu by following this recipe)
- 1 teaspoon turmeric
- 1 1/2 cups fresh spinach leaves
- 1/2 tablespoon extra virgin olive oil

Preparation

1. Preheat your oven to 425 degrees Fahrenheit.

2. Bake the sweet potato in the microwave until done.

3. Remove the potato from the microwave and peel and discard of the skin. You can also opt to leave the skin on (try this, it would probably be delicious).

4. In a small bowl, use a hand mixer on low-medium speed to mix together the sweet potato, almond milk, vegan butter, 1/2 teaspoon of sea salt and 1/2 teaspoon of ground black pepper.

5. Spread the mashed potato mixture on top of the pizza dough, stopping approximately 1/2" from the edges.

6. Heat the coconut oil over medium heat in a skillet.

7. Add in the red onion, garlic, celery, bell pepper, and remaining salt and pepper.

8. Cook the veggies until the celery softens, roughly 5 minutes. Stir frequently.

9. Crumble the tofu into small pieces and add it to the skillet.

10. Stir in the turmeric.

11. Cook the tofu and veggies for 10 minutes, stirring every couple of minutes.

12. Add in the spinach leaves and cook until the leaves wilt, approximately 3-5 minutes.

13. Pour the tofu mixture on top of the pizza and spread it out evenly.

14. Brush the edges of the pizza crust with the olive oil.

15. Bake the pizza in the oven for 12-15 minutes.

16. Remove from the oven, slice it up and serve it warm.

TACOS SIN CARNE

Ingredients

"Meat"

- 1 cup dried textured vegetable protein (tvp)
- 1/2 yellow onion
- 1 cup diced or crushed tomatoes, optional

Seasoning

- 2 Tbsp chili powder
- 1/2 t garlic powder
- 1/2 t onion powder
- 1/2 t cayenne pepper
- 1/2 t oregano
- 1 t paprika

- 1 Tbsp cumin
- salt and pepper to taste

The rest

- lettuce
- tomatoes
- salsa
- any other toppings you love
- taco shells or tortillas

Preparation

1. To do this place 1 part TVP in bowl and cover with 1 part boiling water. Place lid on bowl and let sit for five minutes.

2. While the TVP is re-hydrating, heat up 1 TBSP oil in a pan.

3. Once hot add onion and saute, stirring often, until lightly brown.

4. Once onions are ready add chili, garlic, and onion powder, cayenne, oregano, paprika, and cumin. Stir to coat onion.

5. Add tomatoes. I just use whatever is in my pantry, usually diced tomatoes, and add to taste. The tomatoes add juiciness and flavor but could be omitted all together, in which case add a little extra water when adding TVP to the onion mixture.

6. Add tvp and stir until combined. Let sit simmer for 5 minutes for flavors to soak in.

7. Prepare your toppings.

PASTA WITH FRESH TOMATO SAUCE

Ingredients

- 2 to 2 1/2 pounds fresh ripe tomatoes
- 3 garlic cloves, crushed or minced
- 2 to 3 tablespoons extra-virgin olive oil
- 1/3 cup kalamata olives, halved and pitted (optional)
- 1/2 cup chopped fresh basil leaves
- Salt and freshly ground black pepper
- 12 ounces rotini or other bite-sized pasta

Preparation

1. Coarsely chop the tomatoes and place them in a large bowl.

2. Add the garlic, oil, olives (if using), and basil.

3. Season with salt and pepper to taste. Stir gently to combine.

4. Cover and set aside at room temperature for 20 to 30 minutes to allow flavors to blend, stirring occasionally.

5. Cook the pasta in a large pot of boiling salted water, stirring occasionally until it is al dente.

6. Drain the pasta and transfer to a shallow serving bowl.

7. Add the reserved sauce and toss gently to combine — the hot pasta will slightly warm the sauce.

8. Serve warm or at room temperature.

Printed in Poland
by Amazon Fulfillment
Poland Sp. z o.o., Wrocław